The Best Ketogenic Diet Guide for Beginners

What You MUST Know Before Starting Keto

By: Tammy Jones

Introduction

I want to thank you and congratulate you for downloading the book, *"The Best Ketogenic Diet Guide for Beginners: What You MUST Know Before Starting Keto"*.

This book contains proven steps and strategies on how to effectively adopt a ketogenic diet while being prepared and ready to help your body adapt to this new way of eating.

The ketogenic diet has been around for about 90 years now and was initially used to treat people suffering from epilepsy. The reason why people like this diet is because it helps you lose weight as well (even though it wasn't the initial purpose of this diet). This diet, overall, resembles a state of fasting (where you deprive yourself of eating for spiritual purposes) but where you are still allowed to eat certain foods and also bring to your body certain nutrients. But it doesn't go without issues and that's mainly because a large amount of normal, healthy foods is being cut out of this diet. That is why it is important to educate yourself about this diet before trying it.

We will now go through a list of helpful guidelines that I have put together in order to help prepare for it.

Thanks again for downloading this book, I hope you enjoy it!

Chapter 1-Get Ready to Narrow Down Your List of Foodstuffs

The concept behind the keto diet is to lower your carbs intake in order to indulge in fats. As weird as it may sound, this, in fact, leads to weight loss and has also led to the success of this diet.

Many out there might be very happy with the results that the diet has brought them, but it doesn't come without problems. Not only should you make sure you respect the list of food you must provide yourself with in order to see some results after a while, but you must also watch out for the side effects that come with cutting carbohydrates out of your regular diet.

In this chapter, we will focus more on the kind of food you must look for in terms of nutrition when you follow this diet.

List of food required to see results with the Keto diet:

Even though the keto diet allows you to eat red meat, you'll be pleased to learn that there are lots of vegetables that are recommended in it (just like most classic diets). Note that most of the foodstuffs listed, contain less than 3 grams of net carbs per 100 grams of food, or are simply foodstuffs that contain 3 to 6 grams of net carbs per 100 grams per food. Here's a list below of the type of food you should look forward to buy when starting this diet":

-Your Fresh Produce:

We begin our list with names that might be familiar to you because they've always been considered healthy, like: Lettuce, greens, asparagus, avocados, bok choy, celery, eggplant, herbs, mushrooms, radishes, rapini, zucchini and tomatoes. Added to these produce you can also pick artichokes, broccoli, brussels sprouts, cabbage, cauliflower, cucumbers, fennel, green beans, Jicama, okra, blackberries, raspberries, and snap peas.

-*Your Meats, fish and seafood:*

There are almost no restrictions when it comes to meat, as long as it is unprocessed and grass-fed meat for the most part. You can eat the following types of meat: Beef, chicken, game, lamb, veal, and pork. You can also indulge in meats such as bacon, hot dogs, organ meats and sausages.

When it comes to fish you can eat fatty fish like salmon, as well as white fish. If you like seafood, you can go for crab, lobster, octopus, mussels, scallops, oysters and shrimp.

This diet allows you to indulge in so much meat that you can also indulge in food from your deli counters, such as roast beef, turkey, prosciutto, sliced chorizo, pepperoni, salami, cooked chicken salad, salami, tuna salad or egg salad.

-*Your dairies:* Unlike other diets, there is an extensive list of products you can eat while on this diet. You can indulge in heavy cream, butter, ghee, softer cheese like blue cheese, buffalo cheese, mozzarella cheese, eggs, cottage cheese, and Greek yogurt.

-*Your drinks:* Most of the drinks that are recommended while following this diet are quite light (except for coffee) and count tea (with no sugar), water, and unsweetened coffee.

What to avoid

Although this diet seems bearable because, well, it lets you enjoy your favorite meat and dairy, it also has some restrictions. Since it helps you lose weight, it is perfectly normal that processed foods should be counted out of your list. Also, the keto diet requires eating veggies that grow outside of the ground like the ones we've listed above. So, food such as potatoes, sweet potatoes are to be avoided. Other foods to avoid are bread, pasta, rice, bananas and nuts. You should also avoid high fat sauces such as ketchup, chocolate bars, sodas, fruits juices, donut and beers.

Make sure you draw your list of food and keep it in your bag every time you go grocery shopping. Also note, that you will be required to eat at least 4 meals a day like a normal person. Lastly, if you want a more extensive list of the type of food needed for keto diet do not hesitate to see a nutritionist for more guidance.

Also, keep in mind that favoring organic meat or food is very important here, as you will be consuming a lot of animal fat. To avoid certain diseases, it is important that most of your meat is grass-fed. So, think about budgeting your expenses if you weren't doing it already. It's a whole new lifestyle that you are about to start and preparation through information and getting the right resources is very important here.

What to retain about this chapter:

-The keto diet doesn't cut you from red meat.

-You must avoid foodstuffs with high processed sugar

-More vegetables make the list of food to buy than actual fruits.

Chapter 2-Get Ready to Measure Your Nutrients

Another thing that is sometimes frustrating with the keto diet is that in order to do it right, you have to be specific with your measurements. Which makes sense, because if, for instance, you consume more proteins than fats and healthy carbs altogether, you will certainly not reach the expected results, which is for most people to lose weight and being able to live their lives worry-free. So, here, there's a formula you must follow in order to get it right all the time, and it's all about combining the right amount of healthy carbs, with the right amount of protein, added to the right amount of fats in order to reach the expected result.

So, the big picture (which is losing weight) should be supported by the following formula: % of carbs + % of protein + % of fat = weight loss. Overall, you'll have to master the exact ratios of macronutrients that go in your body (grams of carbs vs grams of fat vs grams of protein.)

Now, let's get down to numbers by giving you the exact ratio per nutrients: You should make sure that your daily calories are made up of 5% of healthy carbs + 15% of protein and, finally 80% of fat.

Let's take an example. Imagine that as a female adult you need about 2000 calories per day. So, how would it work out if you are following the keto diet? It is simple, just follow the rule. So:

- 2000 *5% = 100 calories intake of carbs

- 2000* 15% = 300 calorie intake of protein

- 2000 * 80%=1600 calorie intake of fat.

You must admit that this diet allows you to eat a lot of fat, which according to Doctor Diana Lehner-Gulotta (RDAN, CNSC) a ketogenic and neurology dietician at the University of Virginia, this suppression in vegetables, and especially fruits in order to favor large amounts of fat can lead to lipid abnormalities (which we will discuss in one of our next chapters).

An easy way to get used to this portioning constraint:

An easy way to get used to measuring your intake in carbs, protein, and fats is to use the portioning technique with your plate (that is the plate you will use to eat your meals). Use your utensils like forks, knives or again spoons to divide your plate the following way: 5%, 15%, and 80%.

Next, weigh (in grams) just how much should be allocated to each part of the plate, and make sure you use your normal calorie intake per day as a reference to calculate how much should be put there (see how we calculated it on our first section).

The portioning technique will look like a Hussle at the beginning (like during the first 2 weeks of the diet), but after a while, you will not need utensils anymore to have an estimate of the 5% of carbs, 15% of protein and 80% of fat that must go into your body during the day.

Note that these percentages represent what you will be eating during the day (not only meals). So, this is why it is important to write down the list of things you will be eating during the day, as well as the number of meals you can afford to eat during the day (that's if you know that you will be busy during the day.) So, you will measure the 5% of carbs you will use during the day + the 15 % of protein that you will use during the day, etc.

So, have fun creating menus with the list of foodstuffs we gave you earlier, and make sure you measure your nutrients properly, so as to not go over the prescribed amount.

-What to Retain from This Chapter:

-You must learn to measure your food with the keto diet in order to see some results

-With the keto diet, you will always be required to make up an eating plan that has 80% of fat per day.

-For you to get used to the technique you must try proportioning your food with the aid of a plate.

Chapter 3-Get ready For Some Discomfort Right from The Beginning

The fact that the Keto diet requires you to almost saturate your body with fat all day, all by reducing your consumption of sugar, protein, and carbs may have some devastating results in most of us.

As you may know by now, protein is what our body needs the most because it is, by far, the most complete type of nutrient of them all, just because it helps regulate almost everything in your body. So, if you only eat 15% of protein vs 80% of fat every day, your body will enter a state of ketosis, which results in the body being unable to "eat" carbs, but, instead, starts to burn fat for fuel. We've set up a list of discomfort you may notice during the first week of starting this diet in our next section.

You may experience the keto flu

The keto flu is almost immediate for those who are trying the diet for the very first time. And it has the same symptoms as the regular flu, where you might experience the following symptoms:

- A drop in energy level

- Sometimes vomiting and nausea

- Constipation or diarrhea

- Headaches

- Mood swings or irritability

- Dizziness

- Inability to focus or concentrate

- Sugar cravings

- A hard time falling asleep at night.

Now, these symptoms may make it hard for you to even pursue the diet any further, but in order for you to better combat them, you must know why you are feeling weak and perhaps vulnerable to sugar cravings and exposed to mood swings. First, you have to understand that with a reduced intake of carbs your body is forced to burn ketones for energy (what keeps you going throughout the day) instead of glucose. This switch to burning fat for energy is known as ketosis (thus the name of the diet).

But there are ways to fix this problem and we will cover them in our next section.

What to do in order to have a great start:

Like said earlier in this book, if you think that the keto diet is the one you should opt for in order to lose weight and look healthy, then you should get prepared for it. First, you have to know what the keto diet is all about, then, second, you have to know what to do in order to do it right. So, during the first few weeks of starting this program, we'd already said that you will experience flu symptoms (referring to the keto flu). In order to get rid of the flu (because it's not a permanent condition), you'll have to do the following:

-Get between 8 to 10 glasses of spring water every day in order to stay hydrated. Your body will need fluid to do what it does best, which is to get rid of toxins and help the nutrients you are putting in your body do their job.

-If you work out regularly, try to smooth out your routine a little by introducing light exercises like yoga or leisurely biking. You can do a few sessions of yoga disciplines like Hatha Yoga, which is aimed at helping the body get better while doing a few stretching exercises and helping with breathing as well as your blood flow.

-Since you will also get mood swings during the first weeks of the diet, you should try to maintain a balance in electrolytes. Electrolytes are defined as constituents of all living cells, our blood, and any other organic matter. They include Potassium, Calcium, Sodium, Magnesium, and Bicarbonate, just to name a few. Overall, our body needs it to function and with this new diet, your body will go under "shock" because you will no longer consume them at will.

One way to fight this problem would be to eat keto friendly but Potassium rich vegetables like green leafy vegetables and avocados. So, here, eating at least two salads a day is what you should do from the very first day you start with the diet.

Added to eating these vegetables, you can also enhance your mood by having 10 to 15 minutes of sun exposure (not more), which is said to help release endorphins also known as the feel-good hormones. Enough endorphin secretion during the day can help you feel good about yourself and help you fight these states of irritability or mood swings you might end up feeling during the day and that comes with this diet plan.

-Last but not least, try to get just as much sleep as possible. Remember that this diet mimics a fasting state, where you constantly feel the urge to eating sugary food and the only way to get over this is to take naps in order to stop these urges. So, think about taking at least 2 to 3 one-hour naps during the day, and also try to get 8 to 10 hours of sleep maximum every night (try to go to bed early) for the first few weeks of the diet.

Try to minimize the first signs of discomfort during the first days/weeks of the diet if you want it to be successful. Make sure you load your fridge with enough spring/filtered water and the right foodstuffs like vegetables rich in Potassium that are keto friendly. Lastly, have a lot of rest during these first few weeks of the diet plan.

What to retain from this chapter:
-The Keto diet will make you sick on the first days you start it

-You will get symptoms close to those of the flu while on this diet

-You may be tempted to give up on this diet because of the lack of energy and the sugar cravings you will get

-Water, keto friendly vegetables and enough rest can help you fight the keto flu.

Chapter 4- You will Not Lose Weight Overnight

It is important that you pay attention to this particular chapter because it touches the very reason why you wanted to follow this diet in the first place, which is to lose weight above all things. Now, remember that this diet is very different from the classic ones that either encourage you to eat everything but in moderation or tell you to cut off the fat and the sugar to focus more on unprocessed and healthier foodstuffs. So, what these traditional diets do is that by helping you lower your fat and sugar consumption (whether you are simply consuming less of it or totally cutting them off) you see a drastic loss of fat leading to weight loss in record time. Now, with this diet, things are different, where instead of losing weight you will first lose some water, followed by some muscle loss as well. Now, this means that hydration is a must and that you definitely need some adjustments when it comes to the type of sport or workout routine you normally follow.

Now, why will you not lose weight, and why are you losing muscle during the first weeks of this diet? It is simple, since protein and carbs used to be your main sources of energy and help regulate the functioning of your body cells and membranes by reducing their intake the body will go under a state of "shock", where nutrients will not be processed like they are supposed to, thus explaining the loss in muscles during the first weeks.

The second thing is that you are consuming a lot of fat with this diet, so although it doesn't have the same amount of carbs and protein you are used to, you are still storing some amount of fat (a bigger amount than before you started this diet). The water loss is just normal with most diets, but it's riskier here because of the amount of fat you are consuming. So, make sure you stay hydrated throughout the whole process.

What you need to know from this, overall, is that some changes need to be done in order for your body to adjust to your new lifestyle.

-Change your exercise routine

With the loss in water and muscles during the first week, it might be best for you to think about downgrading your exercise routine as you will not have the same muscle faculties anymore (in terms of muscle strength). Remember that some exercises make you sweat a lot and ask for a lot of efforts in order for you to build enough muscles just like you wish to.

Here's a list of a number of suggestions on how you should, perhaps, downgrade your routine into something lighter (since it is still advisable to build muscles during the whole process):

- If you do some weight lifting you should downgrade to aerobics.

-For HIIT workouts or cross fit you should go for the treadmill

-For those who swim as a choice of workout, you can opt for something lighter like Yoga.

These are just examples of what you should look forward to in order to avoid being injured during the process. Remember that adopting a new diet is like adopting a new lifestyle so making the proper adjustments and understanding why you need to do so (here, it is to avoid putting too much strain on the reduced muscle mass and not losing too much additional water through sweating) is very important. The keto diet shouldn't stop you from doing what you like by becoming a health hazard. That's why it is important for you to follow these guidelines carefully.

-Monitor your water intake

At this point, you must have understood the importance of water when it comes to this diet. It will be the first one you will be losing before you see any changes in your weight. But you need it to survive, so once again, some more adjustments need to be done.

To be effective here and balance things between losing water and at the same time staying hydrated no matter what you do during the day, you can monitor your water intake on a daily basis the following way:

- **Morning:** Take one glass of water right when you wake up and before you decide to do anything (like brushing your teeth, taking a shower, etc.) Drink that glass in full at once.

- **Midday:** Take your second glass of water, but this time drink a half-filled glass of water. Drink it all at once, and make sure that it is right before you eat. During your lunch break, you should have another glass of water (this time full) that you will drink slowly with your meal. Remember that fruit juices are not allowed in this diet.

- **Early afternoon:** During the early afternoon and right before late afternoon you should have between 2 to 3 glasses of water. Drink them slowly and make sure there's a one-hour gap between glasses.

- **Late afternoon:** Take one more glass of water before 6 PM.

- **Early evening:** Drink one half-filled glass of water before dinner, then have a full glass of water during dinner.

- **Before bed:** Make sure that there is at least a 2-hour gap between the time you last ate and the time you decide to go to bed. Have a full glass of water before bed. Drink this glass of water all at once, but slowly, allowing the water to go down.

Note that if you work out in the morning, then, your water intake should increase during that period, where you should get at least a glass of water after your workout routine. The same should apply if you work out during the afternoon.

If you want to make it right draw yourself a water monitor that will work like a schedule to follow in order to get just enough water to function during the day and to help you still do the things you like. Use the model we've given you above to help you create one, and make sure you take into consideration your workout routine.

You will start having results in terms of weight loss after a while. Just don't let the loss in muscles and water slow you down, as it is only normal for people who choose this diet for weight loss purposes.

What to retain from this chapter:
-Water consumption is very crucial when it comes to the keto diet

-Your water consumption should be monitored very closely.

-You will start losing water faster than you will start seeing any weight loss with this diet.

-Downgrading your choice of workout routine is also important here, because of the loss in muscles during the first months of trying this diet.

Chapter 5-You Should Consult Your Doctor Before Your Begin

When it comes to the keto diet, one of the first things you should do is consult a doctor to see if this diet is right for you. You have to remember that planning will help you deal with all the difficulties that can push you to think twice before going for this diet. And there are so many questions that only a specialist would be able to answer. Here's a list of reasons why you should consult with your doctor before starting this diet:

1-You may suffer from diabetes or high blood pressure and be taking some medications to treat these conditions: With this diet, you may have more problems adding up to the existing ones like dizziness and risks of low blood sugar.

2-A nutritionist or regular doctor may recommend that you stop the diet if you are required to have a low-sodium diet due to a medical condition. They can also advise you to use the right supplement in order to replace the salt like, for instance, a mineral-rich salt to help you season your food.

3-If you are currently suffering from an eating disorder, then this diet may not be recommended as it will only expose you to full-blown eating disorders, since most people who tend to suffer from eating disorders claim that their condition was triggered by a diet plan in the first place.

4-Lastly, consult your doctor if you want them to track the improvement of the diet. The doctor may ask for a series of blood tests, as well as other monitoring means, which will indicate if the diet is working for you.

Now, since this diet is all about planning, don't just be a puppet that just has to follow suggestions from their doctor, you should ask your own personal questions and have them prepared (written) before you go see your doctor.

Do not be scared or intimidated to ask questions or to even read them from a piece of paper as doctors are always enthusiastic to help because that's why they are there for, in the first place.

Here's a list of questions that will come in handy once you get to see your doctor. These questions more or less cover most concerns regarding this diet:

-How to measure the different nutrients needed for this diet?

-How should you convert a ratio into grams to get it right?

-Can tab water replace filtered or spring water?

-Are there any tools you can use to help you carry out this diet effectively (like, for instance, do you need measuring tools, like a scale?)

-Are meals diversified with this diet?

-Are there any recommended online sources where you can learn how to come up with menus for this specific diet?

-How long does it take before you start seeing some weight loss?

-Does muscle loss mean that you will start feeling/being weak?

-Is the keto diet safe for pregnant women?

-Is the Keto diet safe for breastfeeding mothers?

This is just an example of the questions you may want to ask and that will be very helpful (we believe). You can draw a list with more questions about any concerns or anything you are curious about when it comes to this diet and remember that your doctor is there for you so don't be afraid to ask for any recommendation or advice.

-What to retain from this diet:

-A specialist can really help you in terms of recommendations or resources needed for this type of diet.

-A specialist can also decide to monitor your health while following this diet.

-A specialist will never hold back when it comes to informing his patient regarding this diet.

-Seeing a specialist is recommended if you've ever suffered from an eating disorder before.

Chapter 6-Get Ready to Set Up an Effective Plan

They say that planning is something personal because it has to concord with your lifestyle. But it may happen that yours end up be missing important elements or a few details that may make a huge difference to your plan and, in the end, render the whole process a success. Well, it is the case, when it comes to dieting and it is mostly due to the fact that it is supposed to be a new lifestyle, which, in turn, means that some old habits will need to be dropped in order to adopt new ones.

We will now cover a series of things you will have to look forward to, in order to get better prepared for this diet and get it right.

1-Write down your goals

This is one of the most important things when you start a new diet plan. You have to know what you want to achieve with this diet because there's no need to pursue one if you don't know where it will lead you in the end. So, here you should decide how much weight you want to lose (is it 20, 30, 50 pounds?), and, also decide/evaluate how long you think you should follow the diet before you start seeing results (is it 3, 4, 6, 12 months, or more?). One last question that should come into your mind is whether you will adopt this diet for a short period of time (6 to 12 months or for a number of years), or if you plan on adopting it for more than 2 years. In both cases, see your doctor to know what happens to people who decide to stop the diet after a while and decide to get back on a regular diet (ask about the health risks, the risks of regaining the weight back, the impact on your mood and if there are any other alternatives that can help you keep the weight off permanently.)

2-Get the right resources needed to successfully pursue this diet plan

Whether it's the foodstuffs needed to start this diet plan or even the little accessories you'll need to make it successful (like scales, calculators, and notebooks, etc.) You will also need to budget your money for the success of the diet plan because organic foodstuffs are not cheap. You will also need to do your homework by locating a number of organic food stores nearby and compare their pricing (this is part of budgeting too). What you should also do is draw the list of all foodstuffs required for this diet, keep it somewhere in your home office or your kitchen so you know about all the options at your disposal. Make sure they are properly categorized (see chapter 1 for examples). And, again, if you want an extensive list see your nutritionist for more advice.

3-Downgrade any workout routine to help your body transition from your regular diet plan to the keto diet

Remember in order to make this diet as pleasantly as possible, it is obviously important to limit the risks of injuries and exposure to hazardous conditions out there. As said in previous chapters try to look for lighter alternatives if you are following a rough workout routine. Remember that although you will be losing some muscle mass it doesn't mean that you shouldn't continue on building some. Consult a doctor if you want more advice when it comes to lighter alternatives concerning your workout routine.

4-Draw your water monitoring plan:

Before you start with this diet, as we explained, earlier you must include a water intake plan, which takes into account your exercise routine and the number of meals you have per day. Make sure you memorize it and keep a copy of this schedule in your kitchen. Make sure you drink 8 to 10 glasses of water every day, since hydrating yourself is very important with this diet.

5-Learn to cook keto friendly meals:

Do not anticipate your meals or just make up any dish with the
list of food we've given you at the beginning of this book.
Instead, learn how to "cook keto" by paying attention to details
like seasoning, how to mix different food, dessert ideas, how
long you should cook certain vegetables or how to make sure
you enjoy your food instead of having boring and monotonous
meals all the time. If you can, do some research about the food
you are about to cook, in terms of nutrients, health benefits,
taste, and how they are traditionally cooked. This will help you
learn more about what you put in your body, thus making the
whole process more exciting.

6-Learn to deal with the keto flu

It's better to know first hand what's in store for you once you
start this diet. It's best to distinguish the symptoms and deal
with them than simply misdiagnosing them with fatigue. This
way you know what to do, and in this case, it should be to eat
leafy vegetables and avocados, drinking lots of water, and
getting enough sleep. If you encounter more discomfort than
what we've listed in our previous chapters consult with your
doctor as soon as possible.

7-Learn to plan your doctor's visits

It is important that you see a doctor regularly if you are having
a hard time dealing with the changes brought by the diet. Have
a doctor see you from time to time, if necessary, have them
book you every 2 weeks for a certain period of time, at least
until your body gets used to the diet.

8-Learn to space your meals and eat regularly

Although it is a very different diet (when compared to the
traditional ones) you still have to make sure you eat regular
meals (between 3 to 4 meals per day). Try to space your meals
(have 3 to 4 hours between each meal) and try to keep yourself
busy in order to keep your mind out of the idea of eating food
all the time (this helps with the cravings). To make it easier to
schedule your meals with the aid of an alarm clock that will
help you regulate your meals more effectively.

9-Learn to get as much sleep as possible

Last but not least, you have to make sure you have enough rest throughout the day. If you are the type who stays up all night for any reason whatsoever, you will have to make the proper adjustments to get more sleep at night, as soon as you start this diet. The body needs to regenerate itself, and it can only do that when fully rested. This is important, especially at the beginning of the diet when your body needs to get used to the shift from eating meals high in carbs to one low in carbs and rich in fat. So, when it comes to sleeping, it's all about extending your sleeping hours in order to help the body get used to the diet.

If you have more questions about this diet and its consequences (short-term as well as possible long-term effects) do not hesitate to see a doctor, once again.

-What to retain from this chapter:

-A plan should circle around several points that are crucial for the success of this diet.

-Talking to/seeing a specialist/specialist on a regular basis should also be a part of your preparation plan.

-You must regulate your sleep, the amount of water you drink daily, as well as your meals and how you cook them.

-Making your schedules, meal plans, and your list of foodstuffs visible makes it easier for you to personalize your keto diet plan.

Conclusion

Thank you again for downloading this book!

I hope this book was able to help you to understand what a ketogenic diet is all about. You have to remember that although it was set up nine decades ago to treat epilepsy, it has been popularized a few years ago because of its ability to help people lose weight. Although deemed very controversial, a lot of people are choosing this diet to attain their desired weight.

Note that before you decide to follow this diet you should consult with your doctor to see if this diet is appropriate for you. Added to that, if you are following any kind of treatment or suffer from a certain medical condition think about taking an appointment with your doctor in order to determine if this diet is safe for you.

The next step is to:

-Set up your diet plan by compiling a document with the required foodstuffs for this diet.

-Get the necessary tools that will help you measure your food and respect the dosage that is requested to successfully complete this diet.

- Think about narrowing down your list of foodstuffs for the month.

-Learn to measure the nutrients you put in your body.

-Get ready to fight the keto flu.

-Get prepared to lose a lot more water and muscle mass than with any other diet.

-Get in touch with your doctor as much as possible.

-Set up your diet plan with all the information and recommendation gathered before starting this diet.

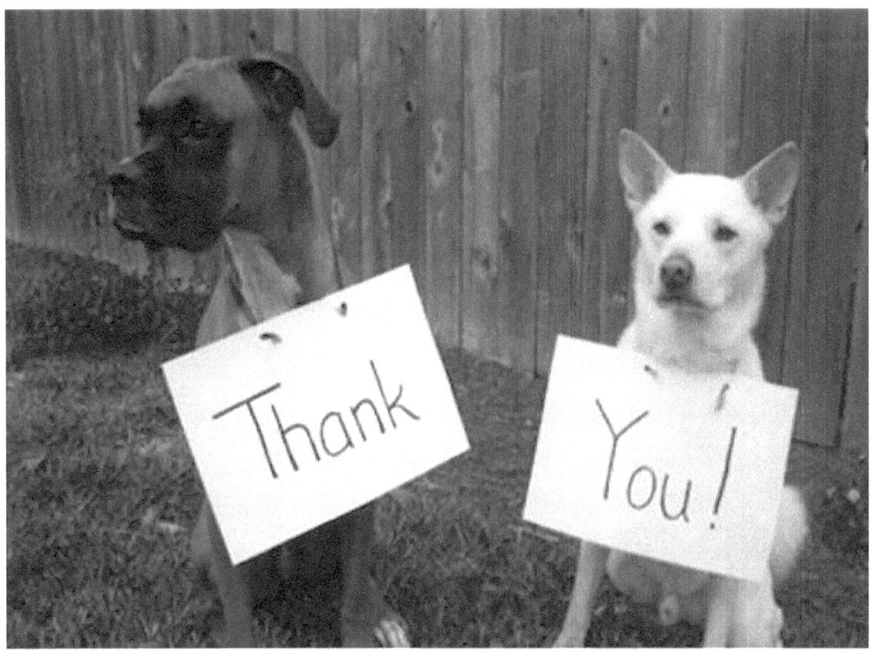

Finally, if you enjoyed this book, then I'd like to ask you for a favor, would you be kind enough to leave a review for this book on Amazon? It'd be greatly appreciated!

Thank you and good luck!